Take Action Now - Multiple Sclerosis

Take Action Now - Multiple Sclerosis

Yoga and Holistic Approach

Dr.Jacob.K

Table of Content

Table of Contents

Description

Multiple Sclerosis is a chronic and progressive disease involving demyelination of the central nervous system which includes the brain and spinal cord. In this book I have compiled some alternative treatments that an individual diagnosed with Multiple Sclerosis can benefit.

Multiple Sclerosis is a complex disease with many psychological aspects. Adjusting successfully to multiple sclerosis requires understanding and addressing these changes along with the physical ones. There are many resources available for education, evaluation and treatment. By using these resources to the fullest, a person with multiple sclerosis and their family can continue to live their day to day life to the best of the quality.

Act now before it is too late.

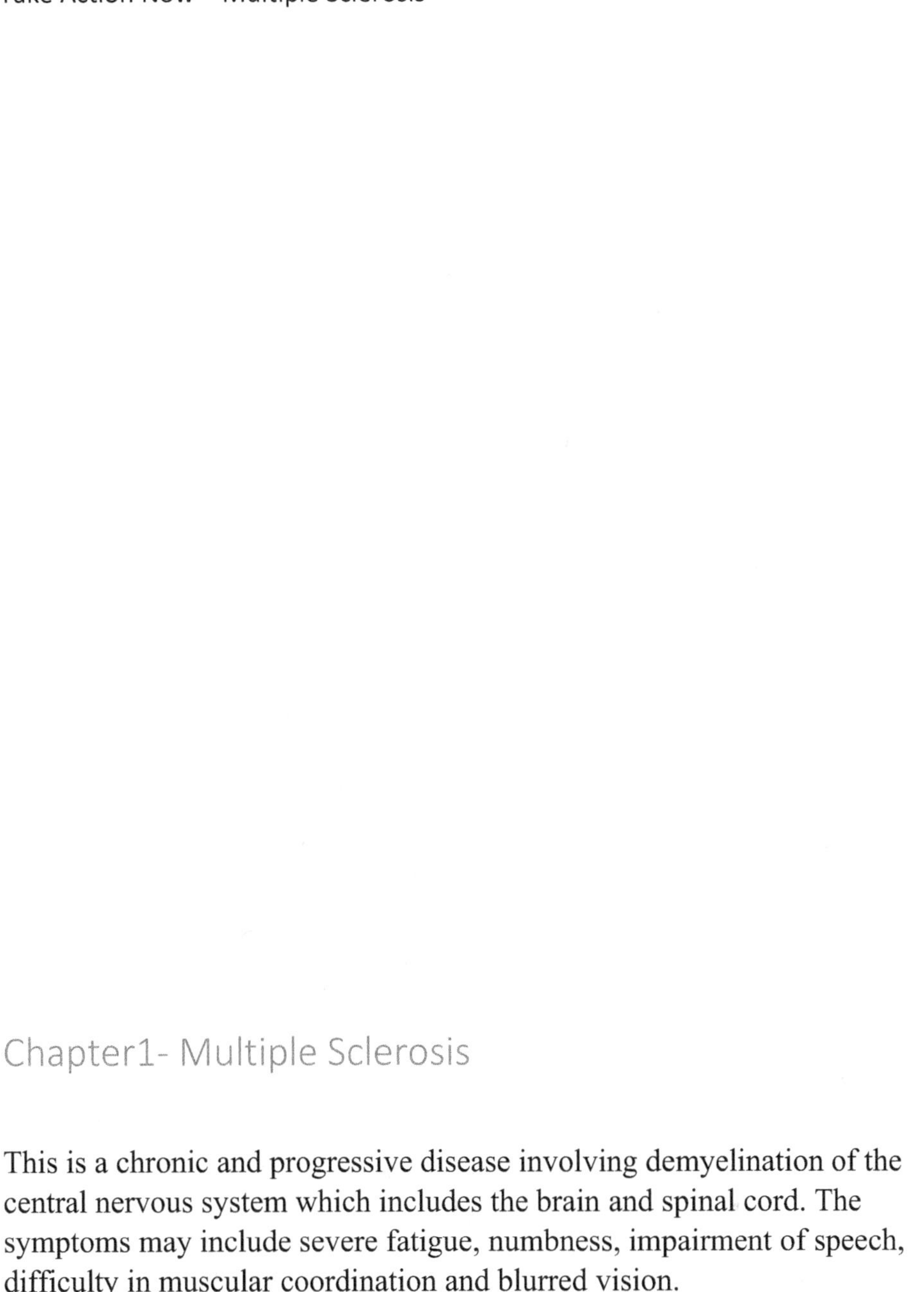

Chapter1- Multiple Sclerosis

This is a chronic and progressive disease involving demyelination of the central nervous system which includes the brain and spinal cord. The symptoms may include severe fatigue, numbness, impairment of speech, difficulty in muscular coordination and blurred vision.

Multiple Sclerosis is a complex disease with many psychological aspects. Adjusting successfully to multiple sclerosis requires understanding and addressing these changes along with the physical ones. There are many resources available for education, evaluation and treatment. By using these resources to the fullest, a person with multiple sclerosis and their family can continue to live their day to day life.

Multiple sclerosis is differentiated from other demyelinating conditions by the multiple attacks that causes lesions to the patients, in due space and time. To confirm such a diagnosis, spinal taps and neurological examinations are conducted. They also review the patient's history to see if they have had relapses. An MRI can show whether and where there have been lesions that injure the brain or spinal cord sheath.

Other demyelinating conditions may result from just one such attack of lesions rather than multiple but can also leave long lasting symptoms. And, as with multiple sclerosis, symptom severity can always vary over a period of time for which we can't say the reason why. The person can have progressive physical disability with muscle wasting over time. Sometimes they will improve significantly, sometimes they won't.

The condition called Neuromyelitis optica it's just a single attack of lesions impacts both the spinal cord and the optic nerve. That how we can characterize Neuromyelitis optica. It can be bit difficult to distinguish it with Multiple Sclerosis as multiple sclerosis can also sometimes affects the optic nerve. So in a nutshell if the attack is just once it's can be termed as neuromyelitis optica and if it's recurrent then it can be termed as multiple sclerosis.

Chapter2. Common early signs of multiple sclerosis

Spasms and Pain - Quality of life and daily activities are challenged for many people with Multiple Sclerosis because of the muscles going into spasm. There are effective holistic treatments and management strategies, including medicines and other therapies that relieve the pain and maintain mobility throughout the body.

A spasm is a sudden contraction of a muscle which may cause a limb to kick out or jerk towards your body.

Spasticity is a symptom of multiple sclerosis that causes your muscles to stiffen, give a sensation of heaviness and difficulty in movements.

Regular assessment of the effects of the symptom and any trigger factors that might be making it worse have to be closely monitored whilst managing the spasticity.

Fatigue or lethargic feeling – Multiple Sclerosis has got two recognised types of fatigue –

Fatigue caused by the nerve damage which can be termed as **primary fatigue**, and the fatigue caused by factors related to multiple sclerosis which is termed as **secondary fatigue**. If you experience fatigue, it could be due to one of these factors, or a combination.

Fatigue might be due to damage in several areas of the brain or spinal cord. It might be caused by the way that the brain adapts to the impact of multiple sclerosis.

The brain tends to finding new routes for messages when the usual nerve paths have been affected. Scans in people who have fatigue show that they use larger areas of the brain to carry out the normal activities than people without fatigue. Finding new routes might mean it takes more energy to carry out an action, and this might cause fatigue.

But there are other processes in the brain and spinal cord that might also have an effect. We don't yet know for sure if there is an exact link between nerve damage and fatigue.

Impaired or loss of Hearing- Hearing loss or deafness is not a common symptom of multiple sclerosis but people can experience problems with hearing. Tinnitus (ringing in the ears) or sudden hearing loss can evolve as a result of multiple sclerosis. Other hearing problems that can occur include the difficulty in understanding speech against a noisy background or being more sensitive to noise (hyperacusis).

Vision problems - Problems with eyesight are common in multiple sclerosis and are often one of the first symptoms people experience.

Chapter3- Associated Problems with Multiple Sclerosis.

Optic neuritis- Optic neuritis is an inflammation that damages the optic nerve, a bundle of nerve fibers that transmits visual information from your eye to your brain. Common symptoms of optic neuritis are pain and temporary vision loss in one eye.

Diplopia or double vision- a disorder of vision where the patient sees two images of a single object.

 Nystagmus- a condition where the eyes move in a more or less rhythmical manner.

Attacks of optic neuritis can include complete loss of sight, partial blind spots (called scotomas), blurred or foggy vision, or colour vision disturbances.

Some people encounters Uhthoff's sign. This condition is characterised by an increase in temperature affecting the individual's vision in some way. This is also known as Uhthoff's phenomenon.

Problems with vision often improve or may disappear after a relapse but they can persist.

Breathing problems- Always keep a track of the pattern you breathe. Mild respiratory weakness can manifest with shallow breathing, which can be fast or slow. This can be missed out at first, as you might just consider it the way you normally breathe. Shallow breathing can make you feel tired and lethargic. Mild breathing problems can contribute to your multiple sclerosis related fatigue and may make you feel as if you lack sleep, even after a proper night's sleep.

Some other common symptoms of mild respiratory impairment may include, shortness of breath, a feeling that one doesn't have enough air, hiccups, cough, and frequent sighing.

Your impaired respiration can contribute to a feeling of discomfort when you lie on your back, prompting you to sit up or change position so you can breathe a little easier. It's an uneasy feeling and always a distress.

You can experience some other symptoms if your MS begins to have a more substantial effect on your respiratory muscles. That can include,

A feel that you are trying to breathe with a blanket over your head

A feel as if you have a heavy weight on your chest or as if you are carrying something heavy on the chest.

Struggle to take a deep breath.

Multiple Sclerosis related swallowing difficulties or inability to clear mucus from your nose or throat may lead to aspiration pneumonia, which can occur when liquid, mucus, and/or food particles enter the lungs and they become infected. It can take a while to recover from aspiration pneumonia, and breathing is often difficult if you have this condition. This could be sometimes a risk factor for the patient.

Speech problems may happen at any stage of multiple sclerosis. Slurred speech is a common symptom you come across. For most people they are relatively mild and manageable. Symptoms may be worse during a relapse or in the more advanced stages of the condition. However, the impact of any changes in speech will be very individual. For example, a mild difficulty could have a large effect on you at work. Or a larger change might not have so much impact on you if you tend to speak with fewer people who know you well.

The most common changes in speech and communication in multiple sclerosis include:

weakness of the chest muscles, making breathing and speech harder, difficulty remembering specific words, slurring of speech, problems with volume, strength or quality of your voice, difficulty following longer or more complex conversations.

People with more advanced multiple sclerosis may find that the rhythm and intonation of their speech are disrupted. They may have slow and fast pattern of rhythms when they speak, perhaps causing them to sound like a robot which is referred to as scanning speech.

Speaking involves several parts of the body that need to work together. This includes the lungs, diaphragm, vocal cords, lips, tongue and nasal cavity. Speech problems can also result from weakness of the chest muscles, affecting breathing and the production of breath to speak with. Speech disorders in multiple sclerosis can be caused by weakness or lack of coordination in the muscles used in speaking. This is called dysarthria.

Damage caused by multiple sclerosis to the areas of the central nervous system that control any of these elements can affect your speech. Similarly, fatigue or weakness can affect any part of the process.

Swallowing difficulty- Swallowing is a complex process starting with jaw and tongue movements, which prepare the solid or liquid (known as the bolus) for transport. Coordination between the tongue and upper throat muscles allows the portion of bolus to be actively moved to the back of the mouth and received by the upper throat. Coordinated contraction of some throat muscles is needed to protect the upper windpipe (larynx), while the relaxation of another muscle allows for the opening of the upper food transport tube (oesophagus). This results in the transfer of the bolus to the oesophagus. From this point, involuntary contraction of the oesophageal smooth muscle moves the bolus down to the stomach, completing the process.

Disorders of the tongue and the throat muscles or their nerve supply will cause swallowing problems. Multiple sclerosis patients may have lesions of the brainstem affecting the direct nerve supply to the tongue and throat muscles. More commonly in my experience, multiple lesions or the multiple sclerosis plaques involving both cerebral hemispheres of the brain cause a lack of coordination of the tongue and throat swallowing muscles. This results in a type of swallowing problem known as pseudobulbar palsy.

For many individuals with multiple sclerosis, altering the consistency of solid food and liquids may be very helpful and improve swallowing function. Retraining to swallow, usually carried out by speech pathologists to ensure advantageous head and neck posture during swallowing, is another useful tool for many people with multiple sclerosis. Other strategies for proper swallowing include: eating smaller, more frequent meals to avoid fatigue while eating; taking smaller bites and chewing these well to reduce the chance of choking; and consciously coordinating breathing with swallowing to reduce the risk of aspiration (inhaling food), which can result in pneumonia.

Tingling and numbness- Paraesthesia is an abnormal skin sensation such as tingling, tickling, prickling, itching, numbness, or burning. In people with multiple sclerosis, nerve damage causes these sensations to occur randomly, most often in the hands, arms, legs, or feet – but occasionally in places such as the mouth or chest. Abnormal sensations may be constant or intermittent and they usually subside on their own. Here are some facts about paraesthesia along with tips on how to cope if the sensations begin to interfere with your quality of life.

As with most multiple sclerosis symptoms, the pattern related to paraesthesia varies from person to person.

The sensations of paraesthesia usually start from feet or hands, and then move up the legs and arms closer to the core. However, they can start anywhere.

 There is no correlation between the sensations and multiple sclerosis progression. In other words, if your numbness and tingling feel worse, this doesn't always mean your multiple sclerosis is getting worse.

 Typically, paraesthesia doesn't directly contribute to the development of a significant disability.

Paraesthesia symptoms can occur with or without a multiple sclerosis relapse. If they come with a relapse, they may linger as residual symptoms. They can last for a long time or for just a little while.

When you become aware of losing sensation (or having abnormal function) in your hands, feet, or ankles, take precautions. Because you may be prone to clumsiness, avoid activities that may be unsafe until the symptoms pass. If you can't feel your feet when you walk, steer clear of rugs and obstacles and stay away from stairs.

These symptoms tend to increase at night and when you're exposed to hot temperatures. If they're keeping you from getting a good night's sleep, ask your doctor for help finding the right solutions.

Stress may also trigger a flare in sensory symptoms. When worries overwhelm you, take a break. De-stress through distraction.

Try complementary and alternative medicine. This help people cope with their sensory problems. Therapies like Reflexology, acupuncture, massages and dietary changes (to minimize foods that seem to exacerbate symptoms) are extremely beneficial. Details of the treatments are mentioned in the later part.

Low levels of vitamin B12, more common in people with multiple sclerosis, could cause sensory symptoms. Get your level checked, just to be sure, and ask your doctor whether taking a supplement might help you.

If you're feeling a burning or tingling sensation in your feet at night, try warming them up if they're cold, or cooling them down if they're hot. Temperature extremes can cause abnormal sensations.

If abnormal sensations are making you miserable or causing pain, and if no treatment strategies are providing relief, consider talking with your doctor about medication. Because medications do not typically eliminate multiple sclerosis related numbness and tingling, they are often a last resort. Like all drugs, they have possible side effects.

 If your sensory symptom is new, much worse than before, or has lasted more than 24 hours, you may be having a relapse.

Lack of balance or dizziness- Many people with multiple sclerosis experience episodes of dizziness, which can make you feel lightheaded or off-balance. Some also have episodes of vertigo. Vertigo is the false sensation of whirling or spinning of yourself or the world around you.

Dizziness and vertigo contribute to balance problems, which are common in people with multiple sclerosis. Ongoing dizziness and vertigo can interfere with daily tasks, increase the risk of falls, and can even become disabling.

Vertigo is an intense sensation of spinning, even if you're not moving. It's similar to what you feel on a twirling amusement park ride. The first time you experience vertigo can be very unsettling, even frightening.

Vertigo may be accompanied by nausea and vomiting. It can continue for hours, or even days. Sometimes, dizziness and vertigo are accompanied by vision problems, tinnitus or hearing loss, or trouble standing or walking.

Bladder problems - Up to 75% of the people with multiple sclerosis may experience bladder problems at some point in their life. Bladder problems are related to lesions that block or delay the transmission of nerve signals in areas of the central nervous system that control the bladder and it is worsened by a patient's reduced mobility.

Bladder problems include problems with storage of urine and problems with emptying it. Some people experience a combination of these issues, which can lead to urinary incontinence. Problems with urine storage make the bladder overactive and include an increased need of urinating (more than eight times a day, and more than twice at night), an immediate urge to empty the bladder, and a feeling of inability to hold the urine. Problems with emptying the bladder include difficulty in starting to urinate and incomplete bladder emptying.

Urinary tract infections are also common in multiple sclerosis.

It can also cause Sexual dysfunction. Sexual arousal begins in the central nervous system, as the brain sends messages to the sexual organs along the nerve pathway in the spinal cord. Multiple sclerosis related changes to these nerve pathways can directly or indirectly impair sexual functioning. The following symptoms can occur as a direct result of myelin breakdown in the spinal cord or brain.

It can decrease the sex drive, altered genital sensations or in other words it can cause numbness, pain and increased sensitivity.

In male difficulty or inability to maintain erection and difficulty in ejaculation.

In female decreased vaginal lubrication and decreased vaginal muscle tone.

Also can have problems having an orgasm.

Erectile dysfunction is a common medical condition which can affect men of any age but is more common in those over 65. Erectile dysfunction may be caused by any number of health or lifestyles factors, including stress, high blood pressure, obesity, diabetes, excessive alcohol use, and certain medications.

By the age of 40, approximately 40 percent of men will be affected by erectile dysfunction irrespective of multiple sclerosis. That rate will increase to nearly

70 percent by the age of 70. The way in which erectile dysfunction affects men can vary and include-

Inconsistent ability to achieve an erection- Around 70 per cent of men with multiple sclerosis experience erectile problems. They generally start some years after the first symptoms of multiple sclerosis appear. Sometimes multiple sclerosis isn't directly to blame, it can be side effects of medication or an unrelated health condition.

Depending on where your nerve damage is, you might find you can get an erection in response to genital stimulation, but not in response to anything else. Sometimes it's the other way round.

Dissatisfaction with size or rigidity of erection

Having erections of short duration

Requiring excessive time and/or stimulation to achieve erection

Cognitive problems- Emotional changes

There are a number of emotional responses that appear to be common as people learn to deal with having multiple sclerosis. Uncertainty, stress and anxiety are the most common, not just during diagnosis, but throughout the course of the disease.

A person with multiple sclerosis may grieve for their life before multiple sclerosis and their self-image may take a while to adjust to having multiple sclerosis. Other emotional changes that may occur in multiple sclerosis include clinical depression, bipolar disorder and mood swings. All of these are more common among people with multiple sclerosis than in the general population. Depression and bipolar disorder require professional attention and the use of effective treatments.

Emotional liability appears to be more common, and possibly more severe, in people with multiple sclerosis. This may include frequent mood changes, for example from happy to sad to angry.

It is believed that the causes are the extra stress brought on by multiple sclerosis as well as neurological changes.

Uncontrollable laughing and crying is a disorder affecting a small proportion of people with multiple sclerosis, and is thought to be caused by multiple sclerosis related changes in the brain.

Cognitive changes

Cognition refers to the "higher" brain functions such as memory and reasoning. About half of all people with multiple sclerosis will not experience any cognitive changes, but for others, the most commonly affected aspects of cognition are to do with memory, attention and concentration, difficulty in finding word, the pace in processing information, abstract reasoning and problem solving, visual spatial abilities, execute functions.

Cognitive changes can have a significant impact on a person's ability to work and fulfil family responsibilities. Family members may not realise that multiple sclerosis can cause cognitive problems and this misunderstanding can result in anger and confusion.

Since multiple sclerosis can affect any part of the brain, almost any cognitive function can be impaired, and symptoms can range from having a mild impact on only one or two aspects through to more pervasive changes, which affect a person's daily life.

Chapter4- Why are seizures common in people with multiple sclerosis?

Seizures may be slightly more common in people with multiple sclerosis than in the general population due to the way multiple sclerosis affects the brain. We now know that multiple sclerosis damages several parts of the brain (the white brain matter, deep grey matter, and cortex), which may lead to disruptions in signal transmission.

The scar tissue or the sclerosis of a multiple sclerosis lesion creates a physical barrier to the transmission of nerve signals down a path.

Types of seizures typically occurring in multiple sclerosis?

Many seizure types can occur in multiple sclerosis:

1. Focal or partial seizures (those that arise from one area or focus of the brain)

2. Focal seizures that generalize to both sides of the brain and cause loss of consciousness

3. Seizures that are generalized from the start

Focal seizures are the most common type in multiple sclerosis, accounting for nearly 3/4th of seizures.

Involuntary and uncontrollable shaking- Tremor is the involuntary, uncontrolled movements of the parts of your body.

It can be experienced as twitching, jerking, or as shaky, trembling movements. Tremor is a common symptom that is found in many neurological conditions, including Parkinson's disease and multiple sclerosis, but it can also run in families unaffected by other underlying conditions. In multiple sclerosis, tremor is usually associated with ataxia, which are problems with co-ordinating body movements.

The most common type of tremor in multiple sclerosis, is intention tremor or cerebellar tremor. This is a tremor that worsens as you use the affected limb, for instance the arm shaking as you reach for an object or try to touch your nose. Some people with multiple sclerosis may experience postural tremor, which occurs when you are maintaining a particular posture, such as sitting upright.

Changes in emotional being- Uncontrollable or out of control displays of emotion are often grouped together under the heading of 'emotional lability' or 'emotionalism'.

If you're experiencing emotionalism, you may find that you have very sudden, intense periods of emotion that seem out of proportion or unrelated to whatever triggered them.

You may easily burst into tears, or suddenly get very angry. These emotions may build up very quickly, and you may have no control over them. The earlier diagnosed the better chance of getting it treated.

Sometimes, these emotions are related to what you're actually feeling. At other times, the emotions you show may not reflect how you're feeling inside: you may react to hearing some bad news by laughing hysterically, or you may start crying when you're feeling happy. Sometimes, you may swing from one to the other with no warning.

Treatment can manage symptoms, but there isn't much we can do yet to prevent demyelination from happening. Based on current research, specialists believe there is a genetic predisposition, and it's thought that a virus or injury sets the lesions into motion. However, the exact cause is unknown.

multiple sclerosis is a combination of things. We don't exactly know what the root cause is.

However, there are medicines to slow progression of disease and prevent new lesions in relapsing forms of multiple sclerosis.

Chapter5- The best alternative therapies to combat multiple sclerosis.

1. Reflexology

Reflexology is a specialized massage applied to the feet and is used as a therapy and as for relaxation. The feet reflect the body's healing forces and these can be stimulated through applied pressure to specific reflex points. It is a systematic practice in which applying some pressure to any particular points on the feet and hands give impacts on the health of related parts of the body. Each point of the pressure acts as the sensors on the feet and hands and is linked with different parts of the body. These sensors will be stimulated by applying the reflexology technique in order to improve the blood and energy circulation throughout the body which gives sense of relaxation, and maintain the homoeostasis. As a result, the body is left feeling revitalised and the normal flow of energy is restored and maintained. Reflexology can be used to treat lot of medical conditions, like depression, anxiety, stress, insomnia, irritable bowel, muscular aches and pains, relieve stress and backache tension. The clearing of energy pathways enables the organs and glands to function properly bestowing a feeling of rejuvenation to the body and mind.

Our feet have got over 7,000 nerve endings. Each foot is worked during a reflexology session which translates into a session rich in communication with your nervous system. The feet have more nerves per square inch than any other part of the body. Reflexology stimulates neural pathways. We've all heard the saying "use it, or lose it" and this applies to neural pathways, as well. The more electrical impulses that travel along a pathway, the stronger that pathway becomes.

Because we wear shoes most of the time, the nerve endings on the bottom of our feet go under-stimulated. Working the feet helps stimulate the nerves so that the pathways remain open to provide key information to the brain about the position of joints, muscle tension and speed of movement. This, in turn, helps us maintain good balance and proper body alignment.
The vagus nerve which is the body's major parasympathetic nerve, is directly affected during a reflexology session thereby slowing heart rate, facilitating digestion, and promoting relaxation.

2. Acupuncture

Use of acupuncture to treat multiple sclerosis is fairly common. Acupuncture is always successful in improving multiple sclerosis related symptoms.
Acupuncture is a technique used to treat pain and relieve discomfort. The needles used in acupuncture are inserted into your body's pressure points to stimulate the nervous system. This releases endorphins, the body's natural painkillers, in the muscles, spine, and brain. This technique changes your body's response to pain. Many people with neuropathy turn to acupuncture to relieve their chronic pain. Acupuncture also stimulates blood flow to restore nerve damage. Any damages of the nerves can be restored with this to certain extent. Acupuncture carries little to no risk.

Although the side effects may include
Pain and bruising. You may experience minor pain or discomfort at needle sites after an acupuncture treatment. You may also have light bleeding.

Injury. If performed improperly, needles could be pushed into the skin too deeply and injure an organ or lung.

Infection. Acupuncture needles are required to be sterile. If a practitioner uses unsterilized needles or reuses old needles, you could be exposed to life-threatening diseases.

Not all people are qualified candidates for acupuncture. Some conditions may cause complications, which includes,

Bleeding disorders- If you are medically diagnosed with a bleeding disorder or are actively taking blood thinners, your needle sites may have difficulty healing.

Pregnancy- If you are pregnant, consult with your doctor prior to pursuing this alternative treatment. Some acupuncture techniques may trigger early labor and premature delivery.

Heart issues- Some acupuncture techniques involve applying heat or electrical impulses to needles sites to stimulate nerves responses can cause a shock to the internal system. If you have a pacemaker, electrical currents may impact the operation of your device.

In addition to acupuncture, you can use home remedies to treat symptoms of any nerve damage.

Regular exercise helps to increase blood circulation throughout the body, specifically the arms and legs. Increased blood circulation can help to restore nerve damage. Exercise can also help to strengthen the body and improve the immune system. Limiting your alcohol intake is very important. Alcohol can increase nerve damage.

Ayurveda

Multiple sclerosis is an inflammatory disease which affects the ability of nerve cells in the brain and spinal cord to communicate with each other. The five elements of nature are deemed present in all humans and notably grouped in three key doshas in Ayurveda – Vatha which can be termed as air or the gases in our body, Pitta which can be represented as the bile or the heat in our body and Kapha which can be denoted as the water or the phlegm in our body.

Vatha is composed of Space and Air, Pitta of Fire and Water and Kapha of Earth and Water.

Multiple Sclerosis is a pathology that involves two doshas – Pitta and Kapha. Pitta as the manager of heat in the body attacks the nerve sheaths (Majjadhatu) that are controlled by Kapha. This disease is usually classified as Kapha roga because the dhatu (tissue) under kapha control is being damaged and ceases to function correctly.

Herbal therapies

Herbal treatments should be given by a qualified person. It is most important in to eliminate stools regularly. Daily elimination is extremely important in the treatment of multiple sclerosis. Shodhana therapies assist in clearing the system. Ayurveda also aims to boost the immune system of the body in order to cease the process of demyelination and counteract the degenerative condition. Therapeutic yoga practised by a master can assist at early stages, however breathing exercises or the pranayama are an invaluable addition to one's daily routine.

YOGA

Doing Sun Salutation regularly helps

Sun salutations are a key part of any vinyasa flow style yoga practice. Many teachers use them as a warm-up at the beginning of class or even base whole classes around them. If you learn this sequence, it will really help you out if you ever want to practice at home, since one of the biggest obstacles to doing yoga on your own is figuring out what to do when you first get on your mat. Sun salutations are the obvious answer.

Breathing

The breath is a very important part of this sequence. Movement from one pose to the next is always done in conjunction with either an inhalation or exhalation of the breath. You can control the pace of the sequence by altering the number of breaths in each pose, just make sure to always move to the next pose on the correct breath.

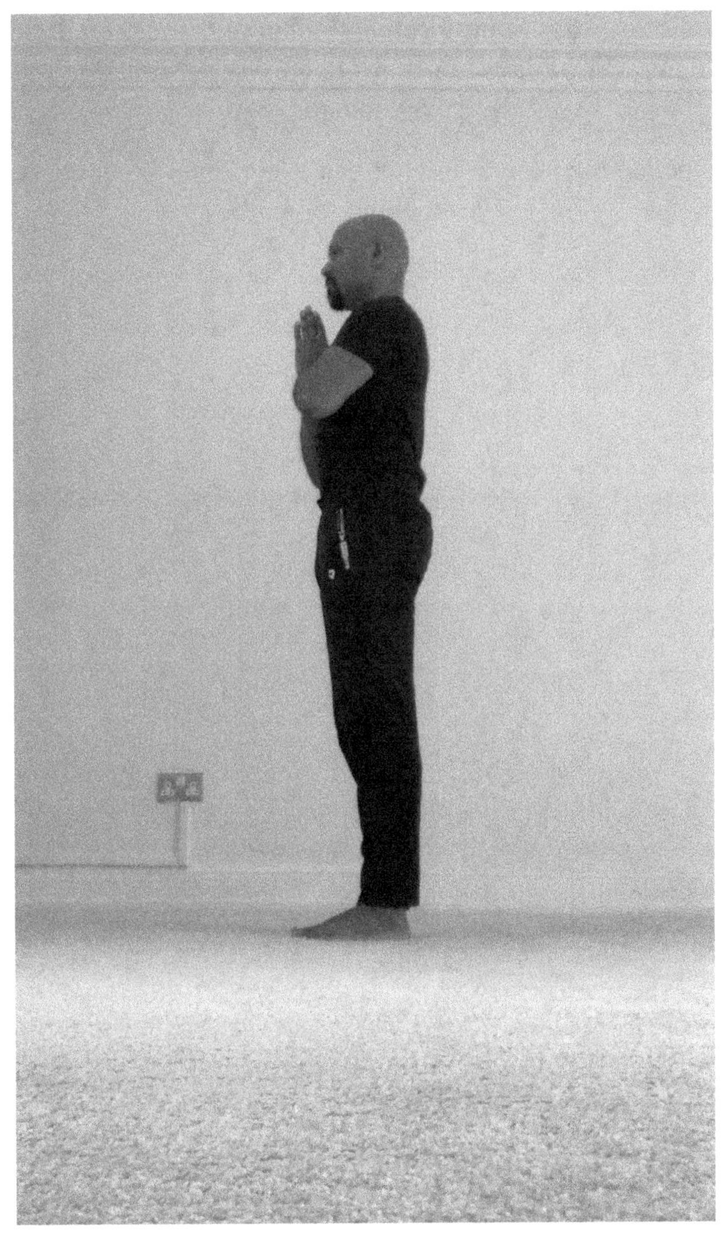

There are various ways of performing the sun salutation. I will be advising you here my way of the 12 postures in the Surya Namaskar or the Sun Salutation.

This is the beginning pose. Join your hands in front of your chest, and your eyes looking forwards.

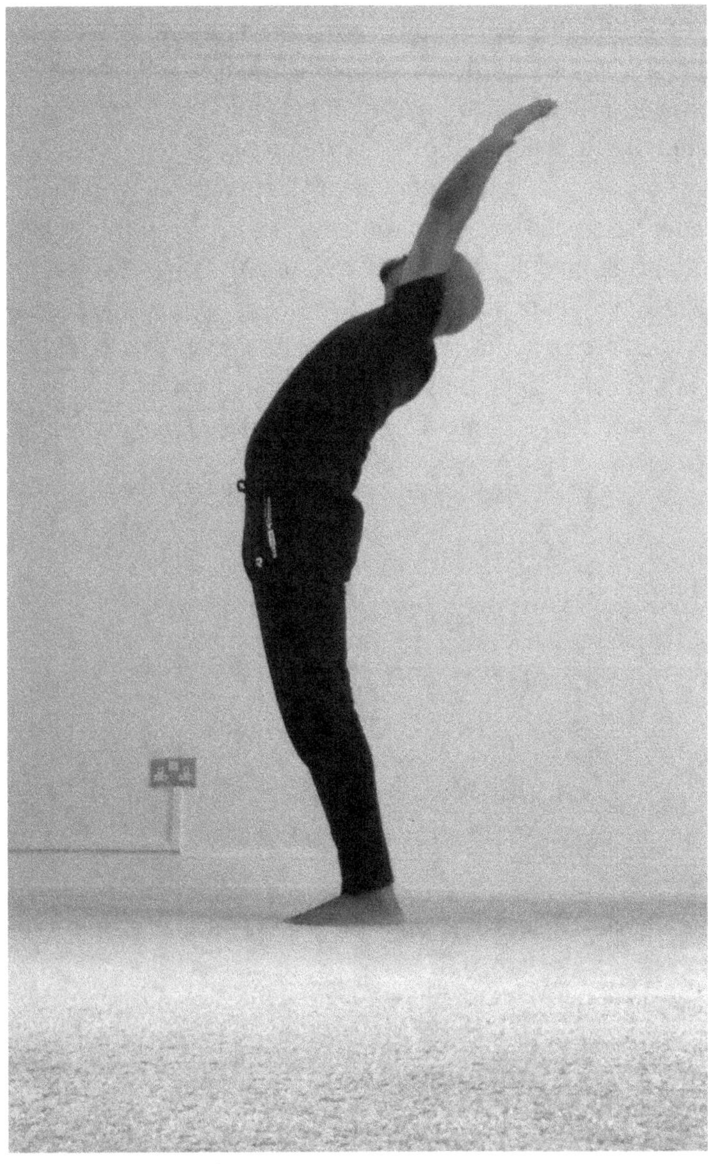

This is the first pose amongst the twelfth posture of the sun salutation.

The backward bent posture. Continuing from the beginning stands, bring your elbows touching the rib cage, slowly move your elbow around the rib cage and bring your elbows together. Now your both elbows and hands are joined to each other. Now slowly move your joined hands and elbows towards the roof, taking a vertical ascend like a rocket. As your elbow reached your forehead slowly drift your elbows apart and bring your hands parallel on either side of the ears. Now slowly curve your back backwards. People with severe back pain need not bend too much to the back rather stay in this posture and do three deep breaths. Three breaths involve three inhale and three exhales. The breath should be slow, deep, long and loud. Don't forget the core muscles are in action when we breathe deep and loud. Volunteering your breath is a crucial aspect in yoga and pranayama. Those who can manage to do the backward bend inhale deeply as you do the backward bent posture. Gaze fixed upwards.

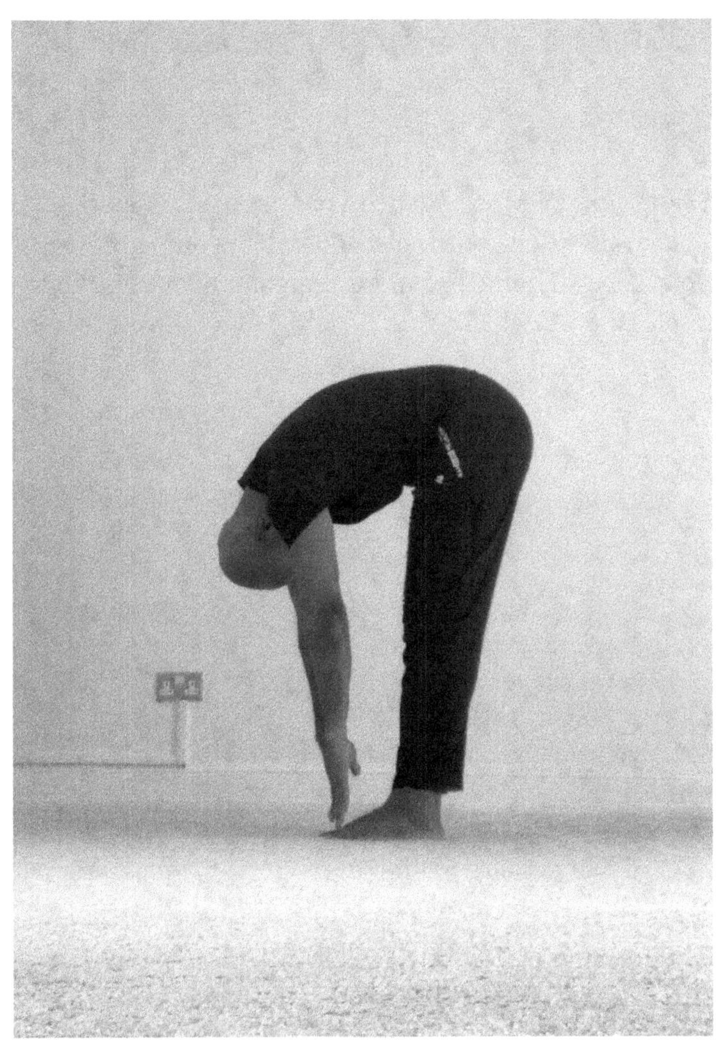

Whilst you do the second posture, exhale and slowly bring your body down, the forward bent posture. When you bring your body down please note that your biceps are close to your ears as you forward bend your head and body, as if you were doing a swan dive into a swimming pool to attain the forward bent pose (uttanasana). Eyes looking straight to your knees. Alternatively, you can keep your palm together and pass them in front of your heart as you fold forward.

Place your fingertips in line with your toes. Flatten your palms if possible. Place your hands on blocks if they don't reach the floor when your legs are straight. Try and keep your knee straight. The more straighter the knees the more the hamstrings muscles are stretched.

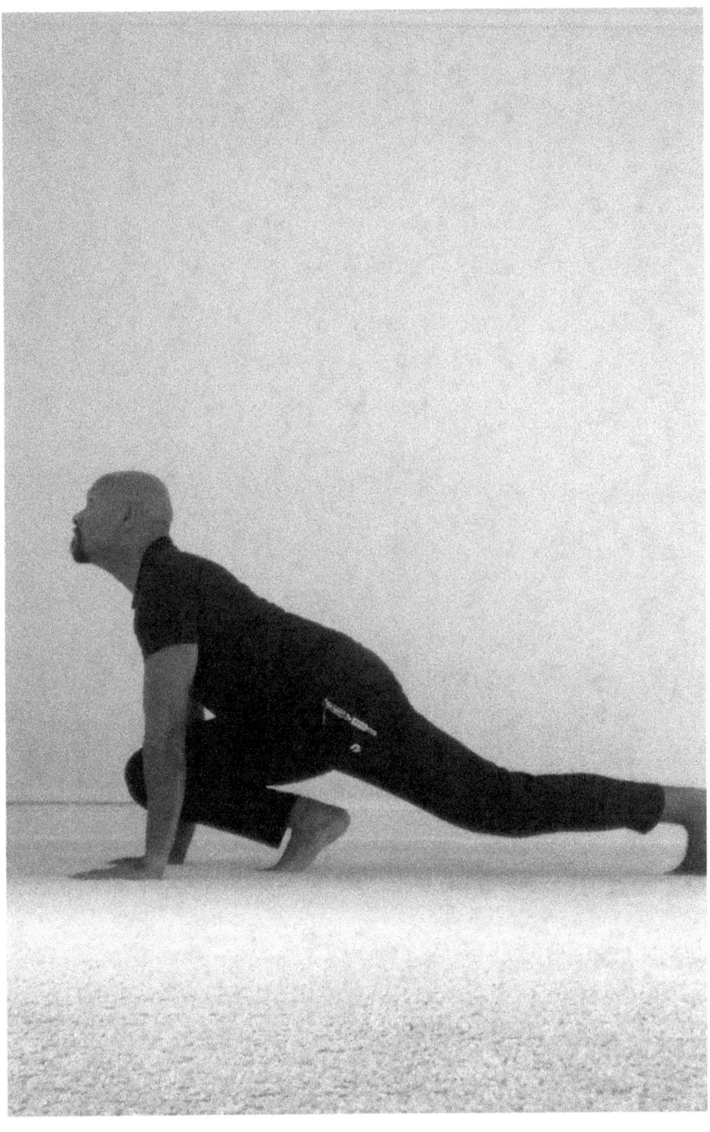

The third posture- slowly sit down in squatting posture, place your hand properly on the floor, finger wide apart and whole palm touching the mat/ floor. Inhale and move your right leg backwards (whilst doing with the right leg), stretch your spine and look upwards to the roof. Please note the hand should not be lifted from the mat as you look upwards.

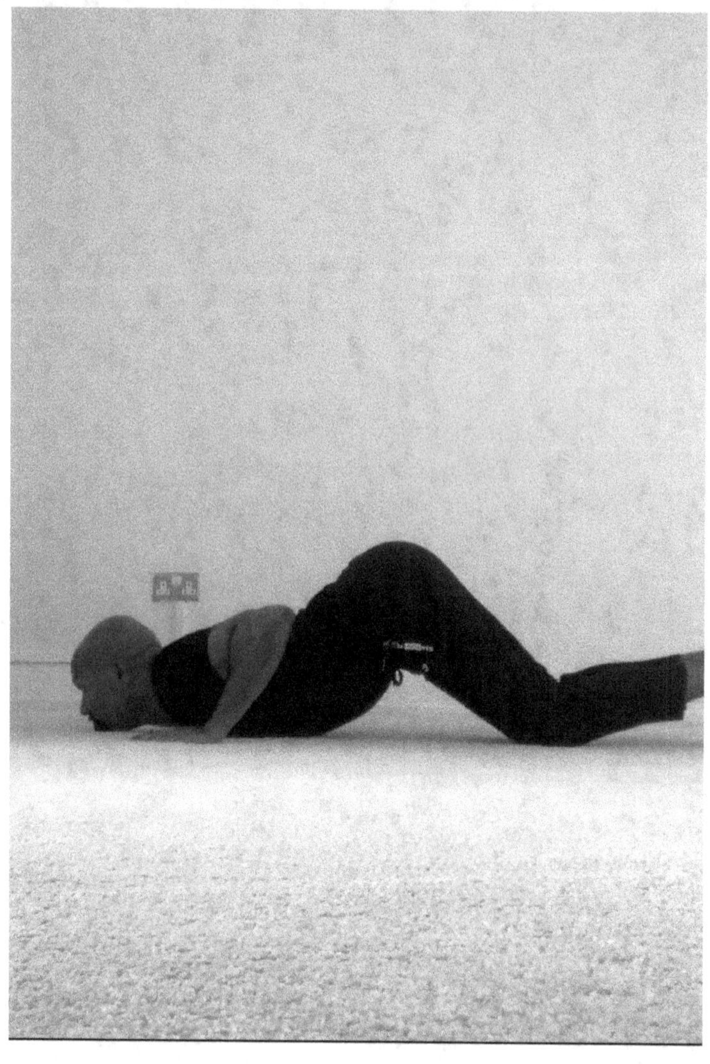

The forth posture- Exhale and now take your both legs backwards, tuck your toes on the mat, bend your knee and knee rested on the mat, your chest touching the mat and chin rested and eyes looking forward. Keep your buttocks high and your elbows hugging your ribs. If you look at the picture above you can see the ankles, knees, hip, neck all angled. The position of your palms are just beneath your shoulders. Palms should not be too narrow neither too wide. It should be exactly your shoulder width.

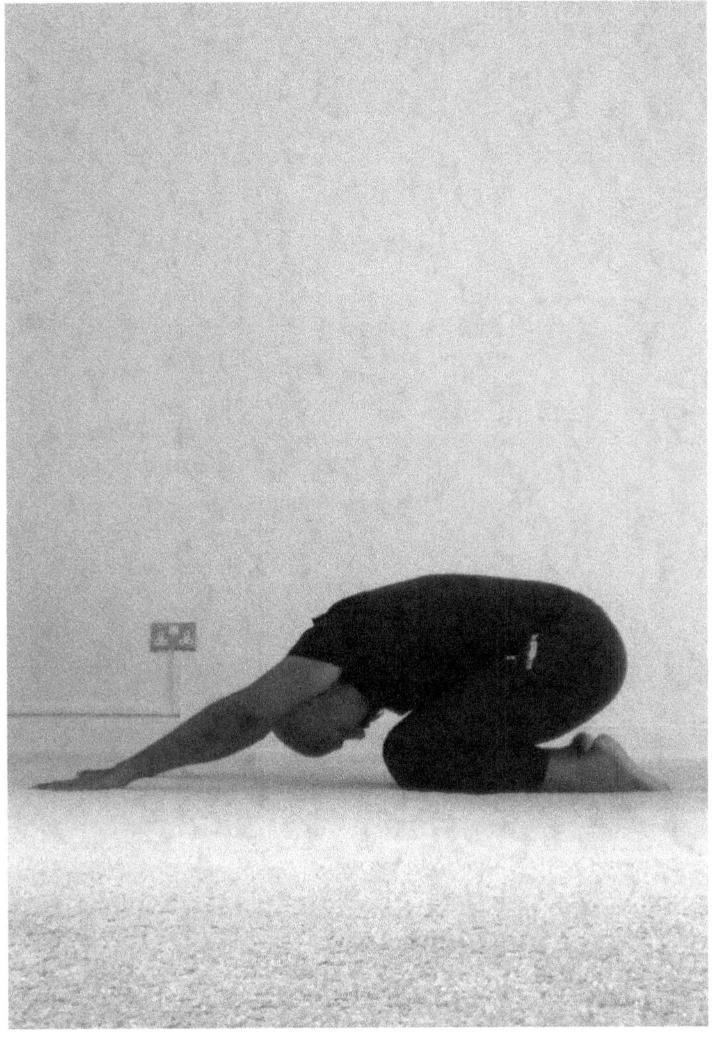

The fifth posture- in this posture you are breathing in and out. From position number four, you are slowly inhaling and pushing your body upward so as your elbows are straight and now the shoulders are just above your palm, which is the four legged posture. Now slowly exhale and slide your body backward sliding your hand on the mat backward and sit on your heels and try and bring your forehead close to the floor. Please note that the spine is all stretched and your elbows are straight. Your eyes looking at your thighs.

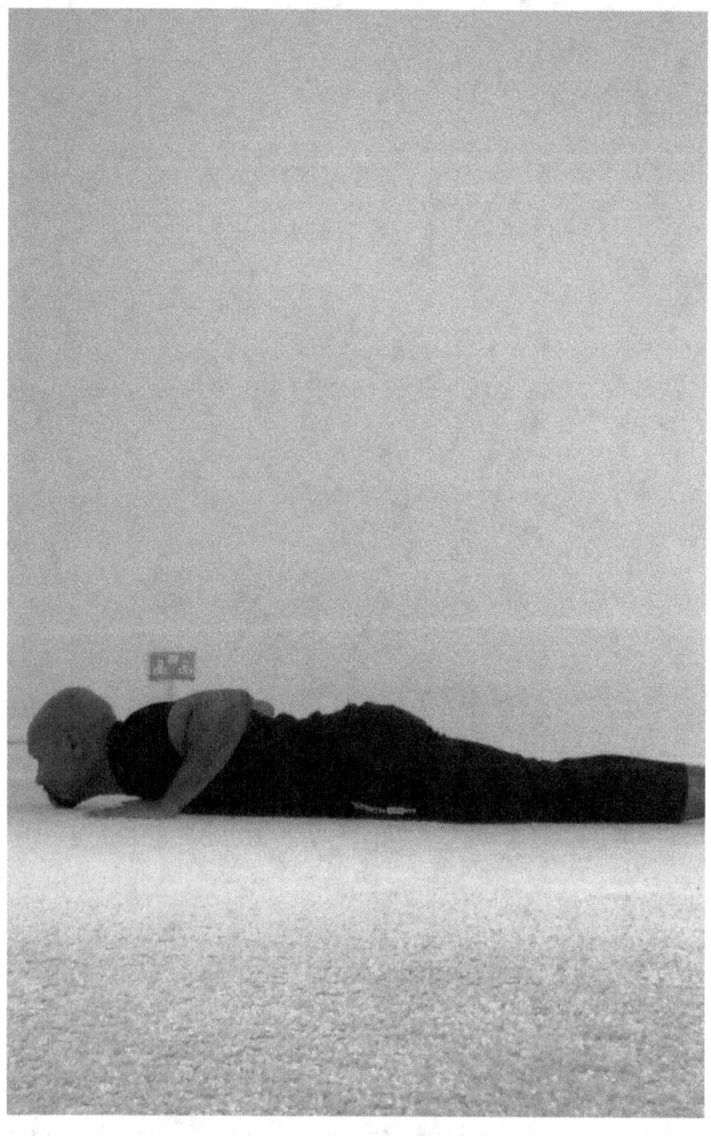

The sixth posture- same like the above posture in this position also you have to inhale and exhale. From the fifth position slowly inhale and lift your body attaining the four legged posture and as you bring your body flat to the mat slowly exhale. Here you are lying flat with your chin rested on the mat. Your eyes looking straight to the wall ahead.

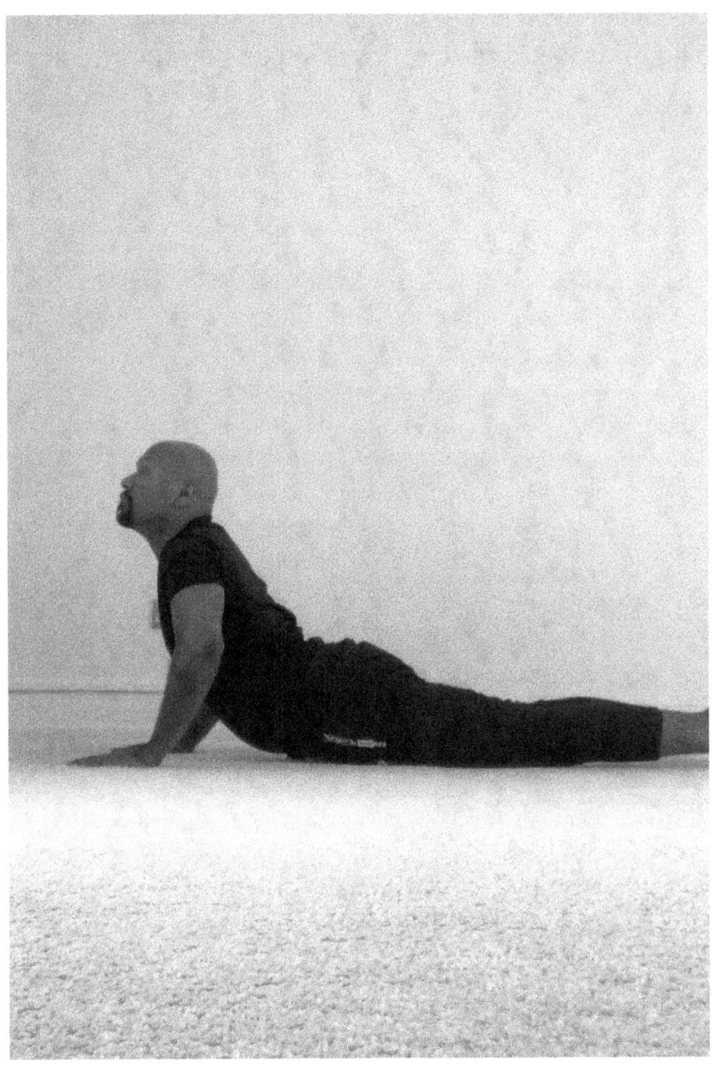

The seventh posture is a very important posture. It's called the cobra posture and it mainly helps to strengthen the lower back muscles. Positioning your palms are very important. Fingers should be apart just below your shoulders and palms placed completely touching the mat. Anchor your pelvis and the top of your feet to the floor. Slowly inhale nice and slow with filling up your tummy. The more you protrude your tummy the more you will feel the tightening of the back muscles. Eyes looking upwards to the ceiling.

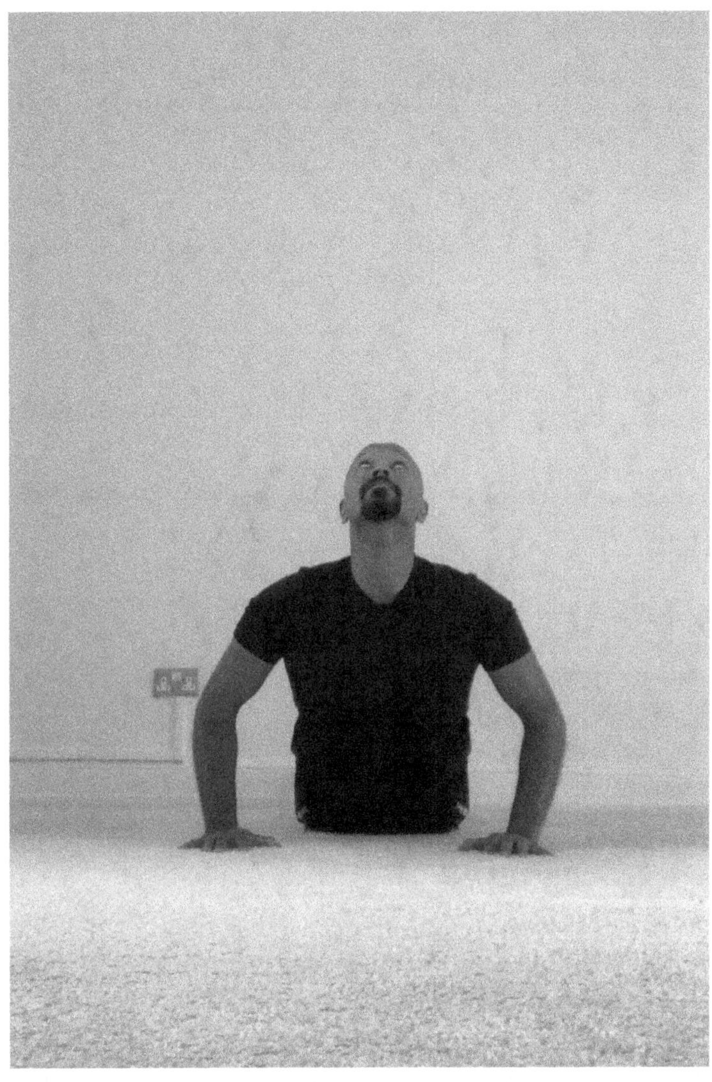

The above image if the front view of the cobra posture. Your hip and toes are touching the floor. Palms should be properly grounded and the back curved. The more you fix your gaze upwards the more strain you feel it on the back of the neck.

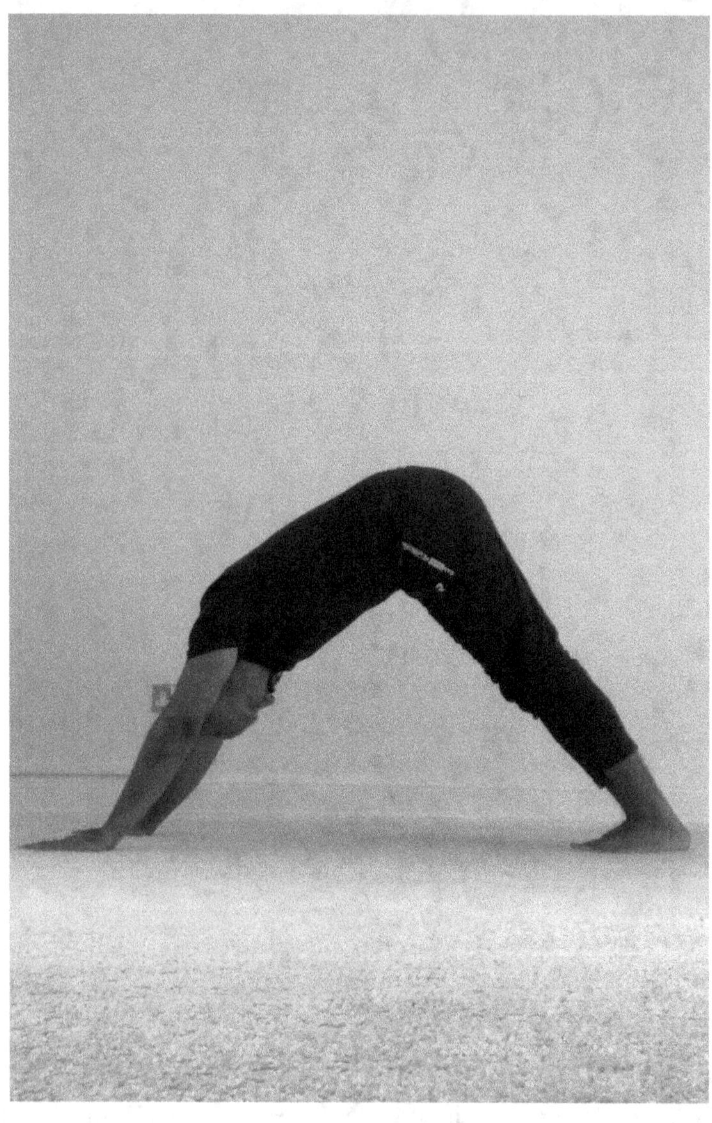

In the eighth posture slowly exhale and push back to downward facing dog.
The right way to do it is, first dorsiflexion of your feet. The feet that was in
flat mode in the seventh posture slowly bring it forwards with your toes
properly tucked in on the mat. Now lift your knees up and then your hip up.
Don't move your palms, they are staying at the same position, just move a feet

distance forwards with your feet and try and bring the heels on the floor. Stretch your elbows out and extend your spine. Keeping the knees straight is very crucial to give your hamstring muscle a stretch. Your eyes are looking at your knees in this position.

Stay here a few breaths (or more) if you need to take a break. If you are going at a brisk pace, just stay one breath.

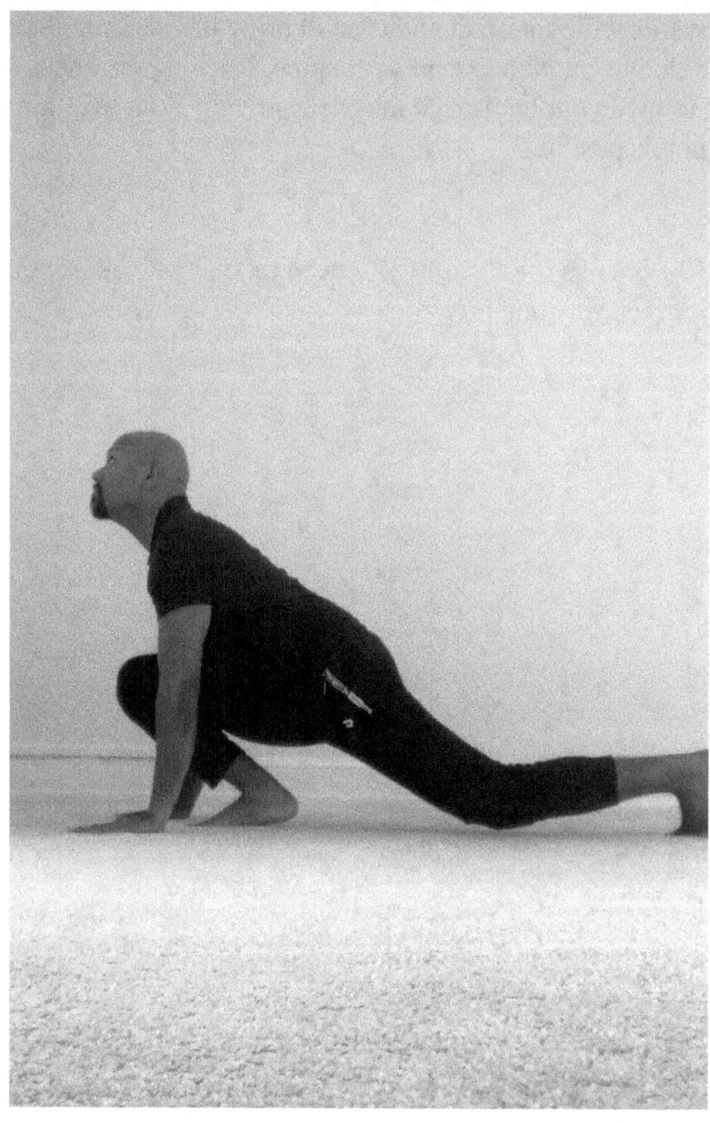

The ninth posture is similar to the third position. After finishing the eighth posture, jump with your right leg in front leaving the left leg at the back (as here we are doing with the right leg). Unlike the third posture here the position of the legs is different. Often practitioners make this mistake with the legs. Place your fingers apart and palms fully rested on the mat and eyes looking upwards. It's an inhale mode you are breathing.

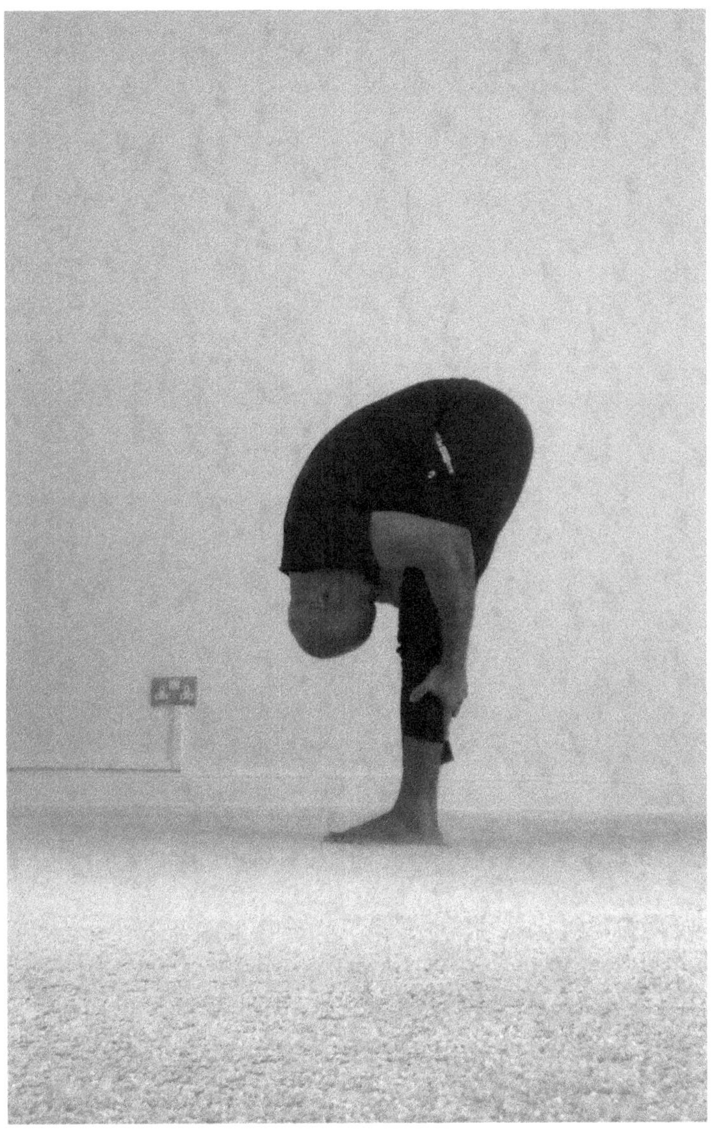

In the tenth posture, the bent leg in front which in our case is the right leg, slowly straighten it and bring your left leg in front alongside your right leg with feet and knees together and hands hanging down with eyes looking at the knees. Whilst attaining the posture slowly exhale with tummy pulled in.

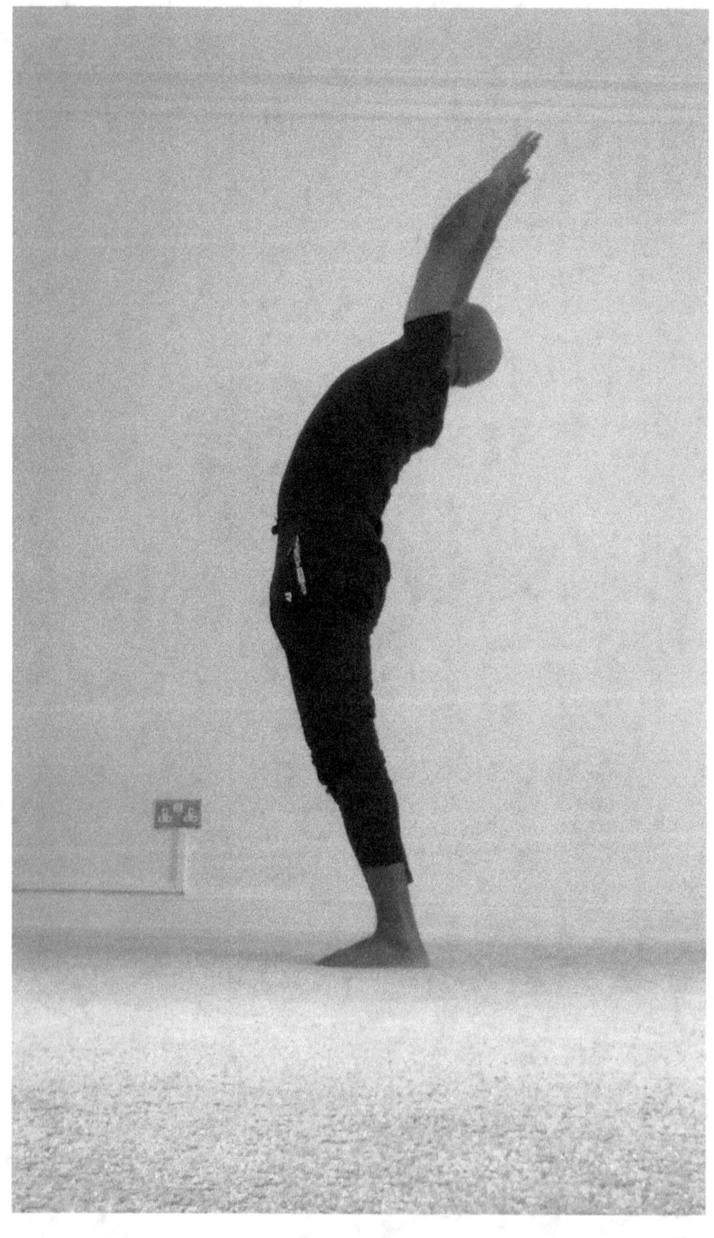

The eleventh posture is the backward bent position. Slowly inhaling keeping your biceps close to your ears bring your body upwards and then backwards giving a proper stretch to the spine and eyes looking upwards.

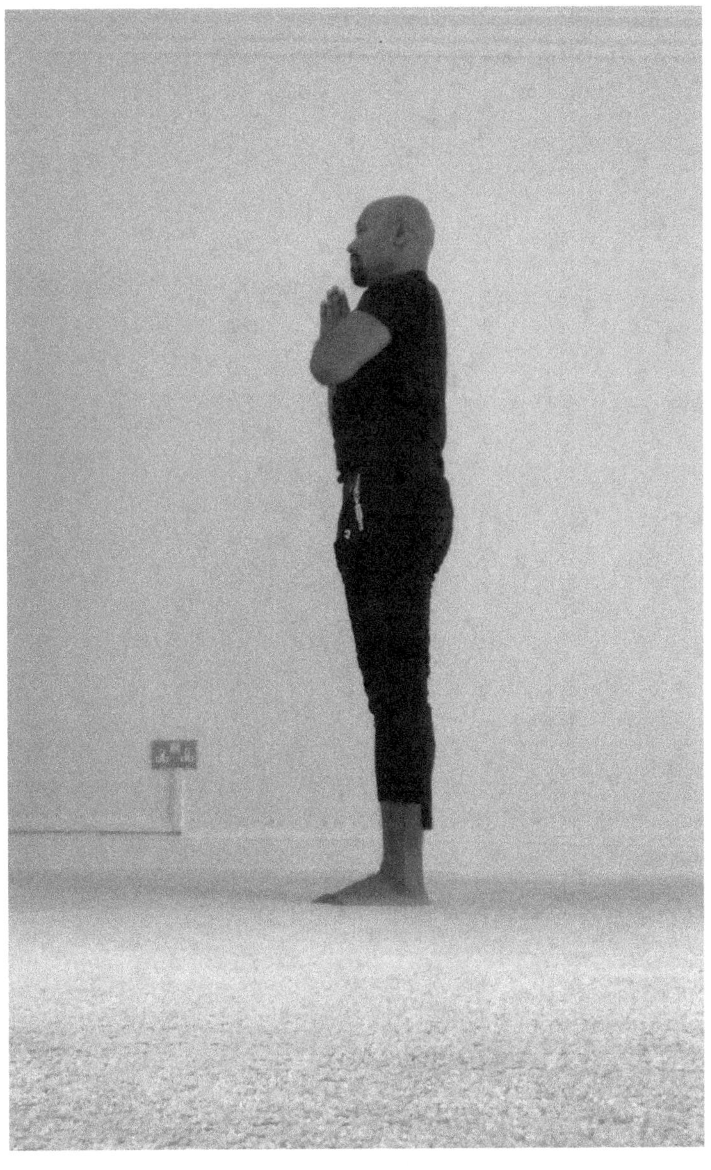

Slowly exhaling attain the twelfth posture by bringing your hands down and to Namaste position from the side of the body keeping your elbows straight.

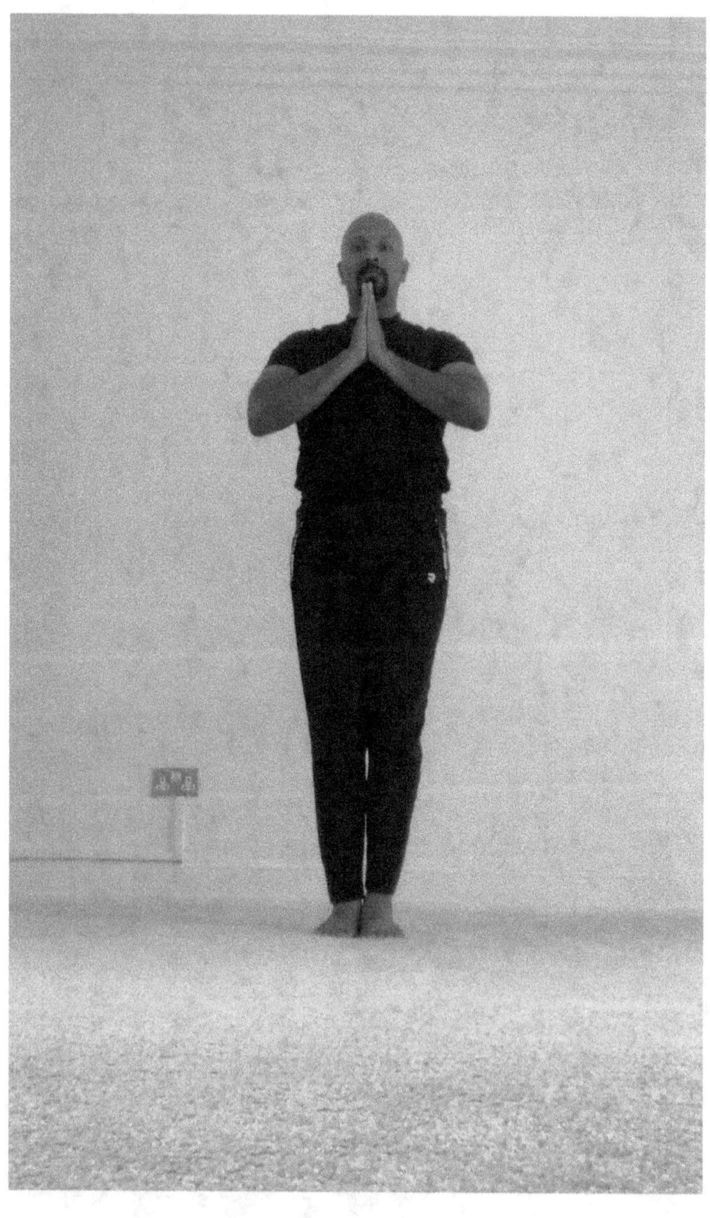

Come to the stands in mountain pose with your hands in a prayer position at the level of your heart.

Chapter 6- Diet & Lifestyle Advice

Though no specific cause has been determined in multiple sclerosis, persons suffering from it often give history of bad lifestyle, addictions, bad food habits, mental stress or contact with hazardous chemicals etc. Rather than curing the disease, preventing it seems achievable. Eating healthy food (mainly vegetarian), maintaining proper food timings and sleep timings, doing regular physical exercises, managing mental stresses properly, avoiding addictions seem to help a lot. Focus should be paid towards the nervous system. Doing yoga, pranayama and meditation prove useful for the health of nervous system. Eating food articles which nourish the nervous system like almond, walnut etc. may also prove beneficial.

Refrain from coffee, colas or soft drinks (sweet carbonated beverages), Cigarettes (abrupt stopping can cause a relapse), alcohol, eating between meals or over eating, too much sweets and chocolate If you like to eat sweets, then eat them after the mid-day meal when they will do the less damage and it digest quickly. Try to avoid fermented foods, acidic foods and peanuts.

Consume in moderation

Black or green tea can be taken up to 200 ml per day, not more.

Small amounts of red wine can be taken – not more than 200ml per week.

Add to your intake

Ginger tea plus digestive spices to increase Agni (digestive capacity).

Spelt (grain),

Whole Grains (wheat, etc.),

Almonds,

Spirulina,

Chlorella, and

Ghee which is the clarified butter.

 One important thing to remember always develop a routine for eating, sleeping and working.

Some suggestions-

1.   Wake Up Early in the Morning.

2.   Clean the Face, Mouth, Teeth and Eyes.

3.   Drink a glass of room temperature water.

4.   Emptying your bowels and bladder.

5.   Rub warm sesame oil over the head and body. A couple of drops of sesame oil in each nostril.

6.   Regular exercise, especially yoga, improves circulation, strength, and endurance.

7.   Do 10 minutes of breathing exercise – alternate nostril breathing is best, but watching the breath pass the entrance of the nostrils is good enough.

8.   Bathing is cleansing and refreshing.

9.   Dressing -Wearing clean clothes uplifts and brings beauty and virtue.

10. Have a hot drink (ginger tea, etc.)

11. Eat breakfast – warm food in small amounts if you are not hungry. Warm food in fairly good amount if you are hungry.

12. Go to work or other daily activity.

13. Mid-day – stop and eat lunch. Eat warm food if possible. Avoid cold raw foods as the only lunch. Salads can be eaten after a warm meal. Take at least 30 to 60 minutes break at mid-day. This should be a main meal in your day.

14. Return to work or other daily activity.

15. Have a hot drink in the late afternoon - 4pm

16. Avoid sweets or candy bars.

17. Return home after work.

18. Eat the evening meal earlier rather than later. You need to have 3 hours of time to digest your dinner before going to sleep. Avoid dairy products at night. No yogurt or creamy foods. Eat lighter than at mid-day. No desert or snacks after eating.

19. Sit 10 minutes and do the breathing exercise that you did in the morning.

20. Before sleep apply a little sesame oil to the bottom of your feet.

21. Cover them with socks and go to bed.

22. You should be in bed by 11pm.

23. Sleep at least 7 to 8 hours.

Diet should be nourishing but simple. Eat enough that you are not hungry at 11pm but not too much that you feel heavy, a strict diet of no animal products and no stimulants.

Chapter 7- Best herbs and supplements for multiple sclerosis.

The below mentioned offers a brief summary of the important information about each of the most common herbs and supplements used by people with multiple sclerosis.

Agrimonia

Agrimonia contains beneficial active compounds including catechin - a water soluble polyphenol and antioxidant and thiamine - a water soluble B vitamin. It also contains quercetin an antioxidant and anti-inflammatory that is also the source of its yellow pigmentation. Agrimony contains the complex polyphenol tannin. This bitter plant compound is a natural astringent. Also present in agrimony are palmitic, silicic, and ursolic acids. Palmitic acid is one of the most common saturated fatty acids in both animals and plants. It's found that palmitic acid may help fight skin cancer. Silicic acid is a compound of hydrogen, oxygen, and silicon that has been shown to be beneficial to hair, skin, and nails. Ursolic acid is a pentacyclic triterpenoid found in many herbs and fruits that acts as a diuretic and anti-inflammatory. Current use of agrimony is based on centuries of its use in treating a variety of health problems. Although different medicinal properties are attributed to the many different varieties of agrimonia. They have the properties of antiviral, anti-oxidative, anti-inflammatory, and boosting the metabolism.

Amalaki

Amalaki is commonly used to promote longevity in Ayurveda. It's also used by Ayurvedic practitioners to improve the health of the blood, bones, digestive system, liver, and skin.

Additionally, amalaki is said to possess cooling properties that can help soothe pitta (one of the three doshas). According to the principles of Ayurveda, excess pitta can contribute to inflammation, difficulty sleeping, skin problems, gastrointestinal disorders, and stress-related issues such as high blood pressure. Amalaki also help to reduce inflammation, alleviate pain, sharpen memory, and protect against cancer.

Haritaki

Haritaki is one of three dried fruits that make up the ayurvedic formula Triphala. It's available in powder or dietary supplement form, its bitter in taste and its rich in vitamin C and substances found to have antioxidant and anti-inflammatory effects. People use haritaki to promote healing from a number of conditions ranging from sore throat to allergies, as well as to improve digestive issues such as constipation and indigestion. In Ayurveda, haritaki is said to support the "Vatha" dosha.

Indian Ginseng or Ashwagandha

This Ayurvedic herb is known by many names, including Withania somnifera, Indian ginseng, and asana. Its berries, roots, and extracts are sometimes used for chronic pain, fatigue, inflammation, stress relief, and anxiety.

Astragali

Astragali is recommended for the common cold, upper respiratory infections, seasonal allergies, swine flu, fibromyalgia, anaemia, in any auto immune diseases, and to strengthen and regulate the immune system. It is also used for chronic fatigue syndrome, kidney disease, diabetes, and high blood pressure. Astragali is also administered for angina, asthma, irregular menstruation (amenorrhea), menopausal symptoms, and beta-thalassemia, and to improve athletic performance and weight loss. It can be used as a general tonic, to protect the liver, and to fight bacteria and viruses. It is also used for hepatitis B, and to prevent and reduce side effects associated with cancer treatment. Astragali is commonly used in combination with other herbs. It is used orally for treating breast cancer, cervical cancer, and lung cancer. Astragali is sometimes applied to the skin to increase blood flow to the area and to speed wound healing. It's also effective for chest pain, side effects of cancer treatment, heart failure, hearing loss, diabetes, heart attacks, heart infections, kidney failure.

Berberis

Berberis vulgaris or Barberry, has long been used in Indian and Middle Eastern medicine for easing inflammation, fighting infection, treating diarrhoea, and calming heartburn. It can be used in many forms and may be used to boost the immune system. Barberries are highly nutritious. They are rich in carbs, fibre, and several vitamins and minerals. In particular, the berries are an excellent source of vitamin C, an antioxidant that may help protect against cellular damage, which can lead to heart disease and cancer. Barberries are rich in berberine, a unique plant compound that may be associated with several health benefits.

Berberine is a member of the alkaloid family, a group of compounds known for their therapeutic effects

Studies have shown that it acts as a powerful antioxidant, combating cell damage caused by reactive molecules called free radicals.

Also, berberine may help reduce blood sugar and cholesterol levels, slow the progression of certain cancer cells, fight infections, and have anti-inflammatory effects

Venom of Honeybees

Venom of honeybees is a clear liquid, and treatment of health conditions with the venom of bee stings is called apitherapy (the venom is also known as apitoxin). Unlike many of the other herbs and supplements used to treat multiple sclerosis and its symptoms, bee venom has been specifically studied for its effects on multiple sclerosis in several clinical trials. These human trials were typically small, and there are still too few to know for sure whether venom-derived treatments may be useful for treating multiple sclerosis. Bee pollen, on the other hand, is increasingly used as a dietary supplement. Although its properties are still under investigation, it appears to have antioxidant and antimicrobial abilities. Others claim it is useful in boosting immune system health and fighting chronic conditions. Deadly allergic reactions to bee pollen are possible. People with suspected allergies to bee stings or bee pollen should avoid all treatment options using extracts or products from honeybees.

Some of the added benefits are it relieve inflammation, work as an antioxidant, helps to boost liver health, strengthen the immune system, can be used as a dietary supplement, ease symptoms of menopause, reduces anxiety and stress, speed up the process of healing.

Bilberry or huckleberry

Bilberry, also known as huckleberry, is a relative of the blueberry and can be used for its fruit or leaves. Although it is often used in foods, the berries and leaves can be used to derive plant extracts for supplements and other medicinal uses. This herb was used to treat everything from vision problems and scurvy to diarrhoea and circulation problems. Bilberry is rich in antioxidants and has the potential to improve vision, reduce inflammation, and protect cognitive function.

Few of the benefits of bilberries or bilberry extract are as follows. It helps to strengthens the blood vessels, it's meant to improves the blood circulation throughout the body, it treats diarrhoea, helps in preventing the cell damage, could help in treating retinopathy, it also helps lower blood glucose levels.

Burdock root

Arctium lappa, commonly known as burdock, has been used in traditional Chinese medicine and European medicine for centuries. It had got the ability to promote circulation and reduce inflammation. It is supposed to be a strong antioxidant and have anti-inflammatory abilities. It is proven to be effective in the treatment of cancer, diabetes, skin conditions, and the gastrointestinal system. Severe allergic reactions to burdock are also recorded, so have to be used carefully.

Calcium

Calcium is a crucial mineral for the body's health and proper function. It is a common part of many diets and is a common supplement. Calcium plays an important role in bone health, cardiovascular health, and cancer risk. Proper levels of calcium are important for each and every individual. Vitamin D increases the body's absorption of calcium, and an overdose of calcium can be toxic.

Chamomile

Chamomile has been used for centuries both topically and orally for skin conditions, sleeplessness or anxiety, stomach upset, and gas or diarrhoea. Chamomile a popular remedy for some people with multiple sclerosis. Chamomile offers antioxidant and antibacterial effects, and it is also being studied for its ability to prevent tumour growth and mouth ulcers for cancer patients. It is supposed to be good for patients suffering with multiple sclerosis.

Chyawanprash

Chyawanprash is an herbal tonic commonly used in Ayurvedic medicine. It has got ingredients that promote immune system. Chyawanprash is effective or helpful in managing multiple sclerosis symptoms.

Chyawanprash can be taken as such or mixed with milk or water or even as a spread on breads or can be mixed with cereals. Having with warm milk helps in revitalizing cells. Regular dosage is 2 teaspoons, once or twice daily in the morning and evening for adults and ½ teaspoon daily for children.

Benefits of Chyawanprash are many. Few are mentioned here.

Immune and Stamina Booster

Chyawanprash is a powerful immune booster and aids body in the production of haemoglobin and white blood cells. Amla, the vital component in Chyawanprash detoxifies the body and cleanses the blood, liver, spleen and the lungs. It enhances youthfulness and promotes healthy muscle mass and tones the body.

Respiratory Health

Chyawanprash can do an incredible job in promoting lung power. It nourishes the mucous membrane and helps in maintaining the respiratory passage clean and clear. It is often used as tonic in winter months as it supports natural resistance, gives strength, energy and combat infections by boosting overall health and wellbeing.

Promotes Digestion

Chyawanprash strongly supports the digestion process in a systemic level. In Ayurveda digestion starts with experiencing tastes and chyawanprash has 5 out of the 6 tastes, except salt. An effective carminative, chyawanprash promotes healthy movement of gases and regular elimination of waste. Furthermore, it regulates blood sugar and cholesterol levels in normal range. A great jam in maintaining and stimulating proper metabolism.

Cramp bark

Cramp bark, or Viburnum opulus, is plant bark that is used to treat cramps and spasms. It appears to have antioxidants and anti-cancerous effects that may inhibit the growth of tumours or lesions.

Cranberry

Although cranberry juice and cranberry tablets have long been used to treat the urinary tract infections. Diluted pure cranberry juice, which is high in antioxidants and cranberry tablets may be an easy way to give to multiple sclerosis patients with bladder dysfunction. Complications with this remedy are rare.

Dandelion root and leaf

Dandelion is an herbal remedy for energy improvement and general health, and it can be used for digestive and skin problems too. Dandelion can reduce fatigue and promote immune health. It has antioxidant and anti-inflammatory effects. The plant does appear to have some medicinal properties that might be helpful to individuals with multiple sclerosis symptoms.

Echinacea

Echinacea is available in many forms and has long been used to treat colds and upper respiratory infections. Evidence is mixed as to its ability to prevent and treat colds. For multiple sclerosis patients, the plant's anti-inflammatory potential for the central nervous system and its ability to promote immune cell health is seen beneficial. Some people may be allergic to echinacea and should take great caution with its use, but the herb is typically safe as a temporary supplement.

Elderberry

Elderflower is known by many names, including European elder, Sambucus nigra, and elderberry. The berries and flowers of the elder tree have traditionally been used for skin conditions, infections, colds, fevers, pain, and swelling. The uncooked or unripe berries are toxic, and inappropriate use of the plant can cause diarrhoea and vomiting. Elderflower extracts helps in regulating immune response in the central nervous system. It is said to have a potential in managing multiple sclerosis symptoms.

Fish or cod liver oil

Fish liver oil and cod liver oil are not the same as plain fish oils, which many people take for the omega-3 fatty acids. Liver oils from fish contain omega-3 fatty acids as well as vitamins A and D, which can cause overdose effects in large amounts. Cod liver oil is not as useful as regular fish in the diet for diseases that cause demyelination. However, the vitamin D in cod liver oil may have a protective effect prior to the onset of multiple sclerosis. Vitamin D and the fatty acids found in fish liver and its oils may offer a variety of health benefits from which people with multiple sclerosis are not excluded.

Ginger

Ginger is commonly used to aid in stomach problems, nausea, joint and muscle pain, and diarrhoea. Ginger has long been used for its remarkable flavour and its medicinal purposes. Its said to have anti-inflammatory and neuroprotective potential too. The potential role of ginger in preventing inflammatory problems makes ginger an excellent choice for use in cooking or supplements.

Gingko biloba

Gingko biloba has got the potential to improve memory. Gingko biloba has been used for a wide variety of ailments over the centuries. Gingko extract or supplements are possibly effective for improving thinking and memory difficulties. It also helps in relieving leg pain and overactive nerve responses. It's meant to be good for eye and vision problems, and even reducing dizziness and vertigo.

Ginseng

There are several varieties of ginseng used for medicinal purposes. Most forms of ginseng have some well-supported health benefits. Panax ginseng, for instance, is possibly effective for improving thinking and memory and relieving erectile dysfunction. American ginseng may help prevent respiratory infections, and Siberian ginseng may have antiviral properties that could help fight a cold. Most forms of ginseng also have benefits for diabetics, but all forms carry the risk of allergy and drug interaction. So have to be carefully taken.

Gout Kola

Gout kola is a popular traditional medicine. It has been promoted as an herb that can lengthen life and improve symptoms of eye diseases, swelling and fatigue. Gout kola is believed to be good to relieve any inflammation. Gotu kola has been widely used in treating skin conditions. It is available in a wide variety of forms.

Hawthorn Berry

Hawthorn plants have long been used in medical treatments for heart conditions, such as heart failure or irregular heartbeats. It is also known for its effect on circulation. It is meant to have antitumor and anti-inflammatory properties that could play a role in fighting other diseases.

Chinese Hemp seed

This is used for its sedative properties for a variety of illnesses, is believed to soothe problems of the nervous system. It is known for their role in reducing spasticity, neurodegeneration, and inflammation, hence it is very beneficial in treating symptoms of multiple sclerosis.

Lemongrass

Lemongrass, a widely known plant popular in aromatherapy and asian cooking, has antimicrobial properties. It also has properties that promote sleep and prevent seizures. It is meant to be good to relieve symptoms related to multiple sclerosis.

Liquorice

Liquorice root and its extracts have long been used to treat viral conditions, stomach ulcers, and throat problems. It also helps to reduce inflammation. It may also have some neuroprotective effects. Hence it's meant to be beneficial in stopping the demyelination of the nerves in multiple sclerosis to certain level.

Magnesium

Magnesium is essential for a wide variety of bodily functions. Deficiencies in this mineral can cause weakness, fatigue, tingling, cramps, seizures, muscle contraction, numbness, and personality changes. Some research indicates that magnesium deficiencies may be associated with some of the symptoms of Alzheimer's disease, multiple sclerosis, and a number of other chronic and progressive conditions. Magnesium supplements and a diet containing natural sources of magnesium may be useful for preventing a deficiency that could aggravate symptoms of multiple sclerosis.

Milk thistle

Milk thistle is used as a liver tonic, milk thistle is being studied in the modern age for its impact on liver inflammation and health. The herb is available in a variety of forms like tinctures and supplements.

Mineral oil

Mineral oil is often used to treat constipation and for skin care. Mineral oil is commonly found in cosmetics and laxatives. The use of mineral oil for laxative purposes should not be done for long-term relief. It is possible to overdose on mineral oil; its minerals and vitamins can build up to toxic levels in the body. This oil can also make other gastrointestinal problems worse in some individuals.

Peppermint

Peppermint has long been used topically and in the form of tea or capsules to promote digestive health, fight muscle and nerve pain, relieve headaches, and ease nausea or stress. It is meant to be good in irritable bowel syndrome, so it can be a help to the individuals with multiple sclerosis who have any gastric issue.

Polyunsaturated fatty acids

Polyunsaturated fatty acids can be found naturally in the diet as well as in supplements. Omega-3 and omega-6 fatty acids may be helpful for reducing inflammation and promoting health in a variety of ways. Polyunsaturated fatty acids supplements may reduce the severity and length of multiple sclerosis relapses.

Probiotics

Probiotics are bacteria that are thought to be useful to the body. They are often called "good bacteria" and are similar to the microorganisms found in the human body. Probiotics are available in the form of supplements and yogurts. Probiotics may be useful in avoiding malabsorption of nutrients in people with multiple sclerosis. In general, probiotics have anti-inflammatory properties that may boost immune and neurological health.

Multi mineral and multi vitamin supplements

Although they can be purchased as separate supplements, many supplements combine numerous vitamins and minerals in a single pill or powder. In most cases, it is preferable to obtain as many nutrients as possible from a healthy, balanced diet. However, some health problems make it harder for people to get enough out of food or make it easier to develop deficiencies. There is still disagreement in the scientific community as to the importance of multi minerals or multi vitamins in the prevention of a wide range of health problems and the maintenance of health. Some evidence does suggest that certain varieties of multi mineral and/or multi vitamin supplementation may help prevent eye problems, brain inflammation, neurodegenerative problems, fatigue and cognitive problems, and other health problems. For some individuals with multiple sclerosis, a general multi mineral-multi vitamin supplement may help prevent deficiencies that could worsen symptoms of the disease.

Myrrh

Myrrh has from time immemorial been treasured for its aroma and use in ritual religious ceremonies. It has been used for centuries for its medicinal properties. It was believed to have antiseptic abilities as well as the power to fight diabetes, circulation problems, and rheumatism. It also appears to have useful anti-inflammatory properties for the treatment of health problems.

Oat seed or oat straw

Whole oats are often used to reduce cholesterol and promote cardiovascular health. It's helpful for improving heart health. Oats' are meant to have antioxidant and anti-inflammatory effects in humans. Oat seed is believed to have antifungal properties. Oat straw is believed to be helpful for multiple sclerosis, spasms, depression, and degenerative diseases.

Omega-3 and Omega-6 essential fatty acids

Omega-3 and omega-6 are essential fatty acids, or polyunsaturated fatty acids, that are revered for their potential to promote everything from a healthy cardiovascular system to a healthy brain. The anti-inflammatory and immune-promoting effects of these fats are expected to be a promising option for supplementation in the treatment of multiple sclerosis. These fatty acids can be found naturally in foods.

Red clover

Red clover is a legume that has historically been used to treat respiratory problems, cancers, and menopausal symptoms. It could also help prevent cardiovascular diseases and is meant to relieve the multiple sclerosis symptoms.

Sage

Throughout the ages, sage has been used for more than just its rich herb flavour. Historically, it has been used to treat mouth and throat problems, indigestion, and mental acuity. Sage also have properties that are linked to memory enhancement and improved mood.

Schizandra berry

Schizandra berry is thought to have antiseptic and anti-inflammatory properties. Animal trials suggest it may also have a neuroprotective ability.

Wood Betony

Wood betony, or Stachys lavandulifolia, has traditionally been used as a tea to treat respiratory and digestive problems. Wood betony oil has antimicrobial and antioxidant properties. It also has the potential to fight other disease-causing factors.

Yucca

This plant may have anti-arthritic and anti-inflammatory properties. Yucca also has anti-platelet effects and antioxidant. It has not been well studied for its impact on MS symptoms specifically.

Zinc

Zinc is a mineral that is necessary in small amounts for human health. It is used to boost the immune system, treat eye problems and any skin conditions and even fight viruses and neurodegenerative conditions. Low intake of zinc can be a reason for multiple sclerosis.

Selenium

Selenium is a mineral that is becoming increasingly well understood for its contribution to human health. It has long been used to prevent heart problems and a number of different cancers, although scientific support for selenium's effects is limited. It plays an important role in eye health, immune system health, and a variety of chronic health conditions.

Skullcap

Chinese skullcap is used for a wider variety of health conditions, such as headache, cancer, inflammation, infection, and allergies. American skullcap has traditionally been used to promote sleep, ease anxiety, and treat convulsions. The two varieties of skullcap should be used with caution; both can interact with certain medications and medical conditions.

Slippery elm

Slippery elm has long been used as a treatment for skin problems, gastrointestinal discomforts, coughs, and sore throats.

Soy lecithin

Soy lecithin is found in soybeans; it is rich in choline, which may be linked to better heart and brain health. Soy lecithin may be useful in fighting high levels of cholesterol and in raising choline levels in the brain.

St. John's wort

St. John's wort has traditionally been used for nerve pain, mental health problems like depression and anxiety, and as a balm for wounds. Its impact on depressive symptoms is well known. St. John's wort is starting to be evaluated for its ability to promote the healing and health of nerves.

Stevia

This popular alternative to sugar has long been used for diabetes treatment. It has been also said to have antioxidant effects and other properties that could potentially improve liver and kidney health.

Turmeric

Turmeric is a popular spice containing curcuminoids. Curcuminoids have been shown to have neuroprotective effects. Its anti-inflammatory abilities also show promise for the alleviation of multiple sclerosis symptoms and other autoimmune diseases.

Valerian

Valerian is used for headaches, trembling, and a variety of sleep disorders, valerian has also been used for anxiety and depression. It is meant to be good for insomnia and anxiety.

Vitamin A

This fat-soluble vitamin plays a critical role in vision, reproductive health, and the immune system. Vitamin A is also important for proper function of the heart and other organs. Vitamin A can be found naturally in a variety of foods such as leafy greens, fruits and dairy products or obtained through a supplement. It is possible to overdose on vitamin A, and it should not be taken in large doses. Vitamin A supplementation has been linked to delays in age-related macular degeneration.

Vitamin B-1 (thiamine)

Vitamin B-1, also known as thiamine or thiamin, is essential for proper brain function. Deficiency of vitamin B-1 can also cause weakness and fatigue. Thiamine can be found in nuts, seeds, legumes, whole grains, eggs, and lean meats. Thiamine is also essential for healthy metabolism and nerve, muscle, and heart function. Deficiencies in thiamine are associated with a variety of neurodegenerative conditions including multiple sclerosis.

Vitamin B-6

Vitamin B-6 is an essential nutrient for metabolism that is found in certain foods such as organ meats, fish, and starchy vegetables and supplements. Although deficiencies are rare, low vitamin B-6 levels are not uncommon in autoimmune disorders.

Vitamin B-12

Vitamin B-12 is important for the proper function of nerve cells, red blood cells, the brain, and many other body parts. People with multiple sclerosis may be more likely to develop a B-12 deficiency, making supplementation a good option for some individuals. Together, vitamins B-6 and B-12 may be important for eye health. Deficiencies lead to weakness, weight loss, numbness and tingling in hands and feet, balance problems, confusion, memory problems, and even nerve damage.

Vitamin C

Vitamin C, or ascorbic acid, is an important player in the function of the immune system. It is an antioxidant that may not be absorbed as well by individuals with multiple sclerosis. Although vitamin C deficiencies are rare, they can cause serious problems like depression, tooth loss, fatigue, joint pain, and even death. Ascorbic acid is essential to eye health and the prevention of macular degeneration and cataracts. Vitamin C's antioxidants may help protect individuals with multiple sclerosis from deterioration.

Vitamin D

Vitamin D is essential for bone, muscle, nerve and immune system health. Most people obtain vitamin D from sun exposure, fatty fish, and fortified foods and drinks. Sun exposure and monitored vitamin D supplementation is becoming a more common recommendation for the treatment of multiple sclerosis.

Vitamin E

Vitamin E is an important fat-soluble nutrient and antioxidant. It is essential for immune system health and preventing blood clots. Vegetable oils, nuts, and green vegetables are the best food sources of vitamin E. People with multiple sclerosis may have low levels of vitamin E, so its intake will be helpful.